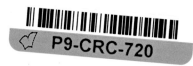

It's Catching

Whooping Cough

Elizabeth Laskey

Designed by Patricia Stevenson
Printed and bound in the United States by Lake Book Manufacturing

07 06 05 04 03
10 9 8 7 6 5 4 3 2 1

Library of Congress Cataloging-in-Publication Data
Laskey, Elizabeth, 1961–
        Whooping cough / Elizabeth Laskey.
             v. cm. — (It's catching)
        Includes bibliographical references and index.
        Contents: What is whooping cough? — Healthy nose, throat, and lungs —
        What causes whooping cough? — How do you catch it? —
        First signs — The whooping stage — Why you cough — Treatment —
        Whooping cough can be dangerous — Getting better —
        Avoiding whooping cough — Staying healthy — Think about it.
        ISBN 1-4034-0277-9
        1. Whooping cough—Juvenile literature. [1. Whooping cough. 2. Diseases.]
        I. Title. II. Series.

        RC204 .L374 2002
        616.2'04—dc21
                                        2001008568

Acknowledgments
The author and publishers are grateful to the following for permission to reproduce copyright material:
Cover photograph by Jack Ballard/Visuals Unlimited
p. 4 Ed Wheeler/Corbis Stock Market; p. 5 O'Brien Productions/Corbis; p. 6 M. Dauenheimer/Custom Medical Stock Photo, Inc.; p. 7 Custom Medical Stock Photo, Inc.; p. 8 Oliver Meckes/Photo Researchers, Inc.; p. 9 Carolyn A. McKeone/Photo Researchers, Inc.; p. 10 David Young-Wolff/PhotoEdit; p. 11 Jeff Greenberg/PhotoEdit/PictureQuest; pp. 12, 16 Edward Lettau/Photo Researchers, Inc.; p. 13 Rob Lewine/Corbis Stock Market; p. 14 NMSB/Custom Medical Stock Photo, Inc.; p. 15 Burger Phanie, Rex Interstock/Stock Connection/PictureQuest; p. 17 Oscar Burriel/Science Photo Library/Photo Researchers, Inc.; pp. 18, 19 Blair Seitz/Photo Researchers, Inc.; p. 20 Jon Feingersh/Corbis Stock Market; p. 21 Kathy Sloane/Photo Researchers, Inc.; p. 22 Peter Fownes/Stock South/PictureQuest; p. 23 Michael Newman/PhotoEdit; p. 24 Saturn Stills/Science Photo Library/Photo Researchers, Inc.; p. 25 Lawrence Migdale/Stock Boston, Inc.; p. 26 Michael A. Keller Studios/Corbis Stock Market; p. 27 Felicia Martinez/PhotoEdit/PictureQuest; p. 28 Laura Dwight/Corbis; p. 29 Merritt Vincent/PhotoEdit
Every effort has been made to contact copyright holders of any material reproduced in this book. Any omissions will be rectified in subsequent printings if notice is given to the publisher.

Some words are shown in bold, **like this.** You can find out what they mean by looking in the glossary.

Contents

What Is Whooping Cough?

Whooping cough is an illness that makes you cough a lot. People with whooping cough sometimes make a "whoop" sound after they cough. This is how the illness got its name.

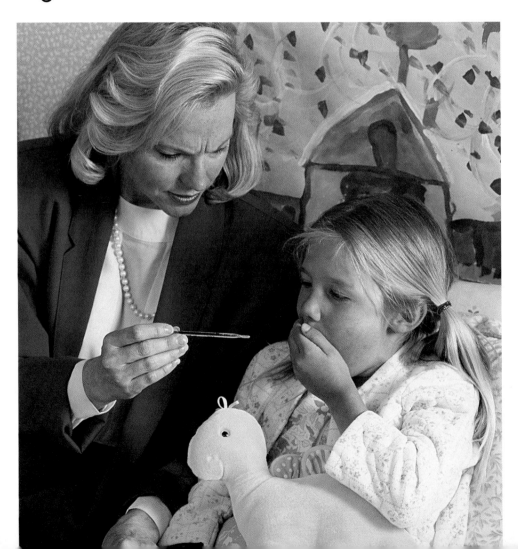

Whooping cough is an **infectious** illness. This means it can spread from one person to another.

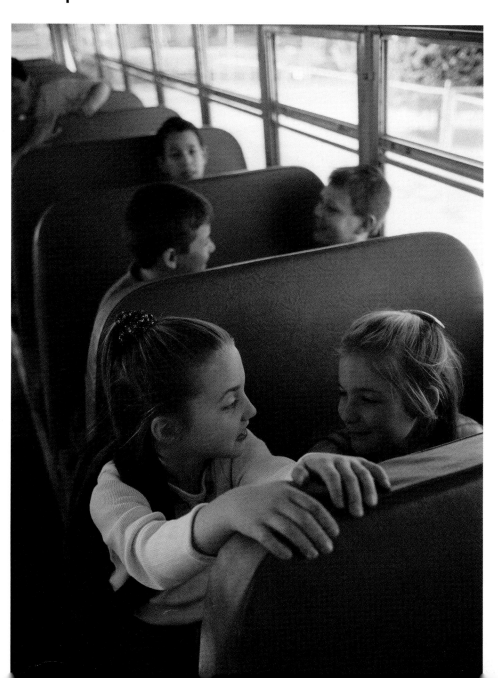

Healthy Nose, Throat, and Lungs

When you breathe, air passes in through your nose, down a part of your throat called the **trachea,** and into your **lungs.**

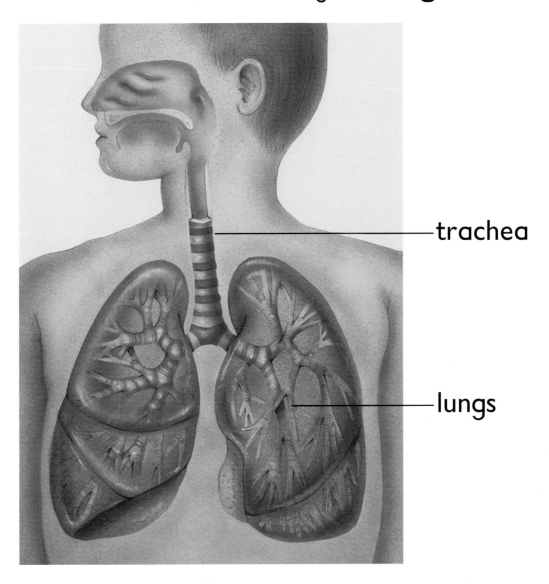

trachea

lungs

The insides of your nose and throat make **mucus.** Mucus is sticky. It traps **germs** that get in through your nose and mouth. This helps keep you from getting sick.

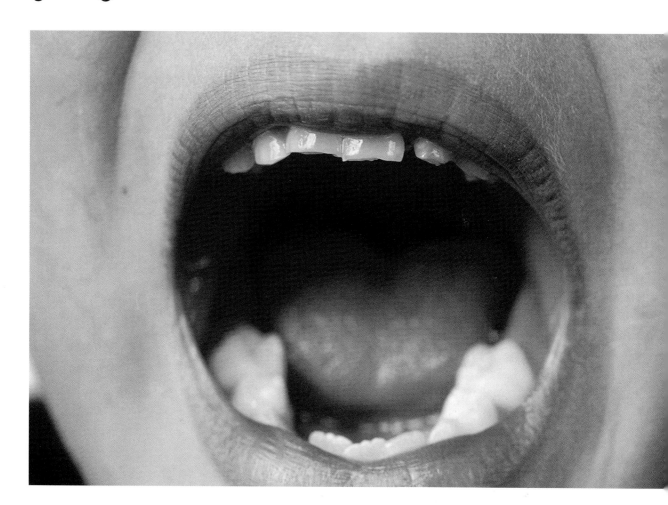

What Causes Whooping Cough?

Whooping cough is caused by **bacteria.**
Bacteria are tiny living things. They are
so small you need a **microscope** to see
them. This is what whooping cough bacteria
look like through a microscope.

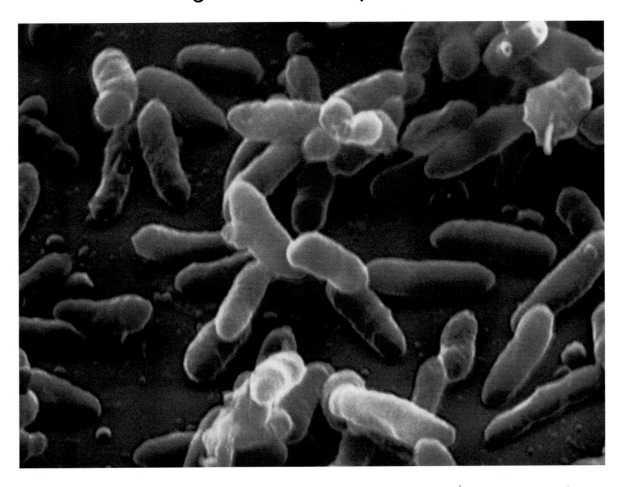

Some bacteria cause **infections** if they get inside your body. If whooping cough bacteria get inside your body, they can make many more bacteria. When this happens, you get sick.

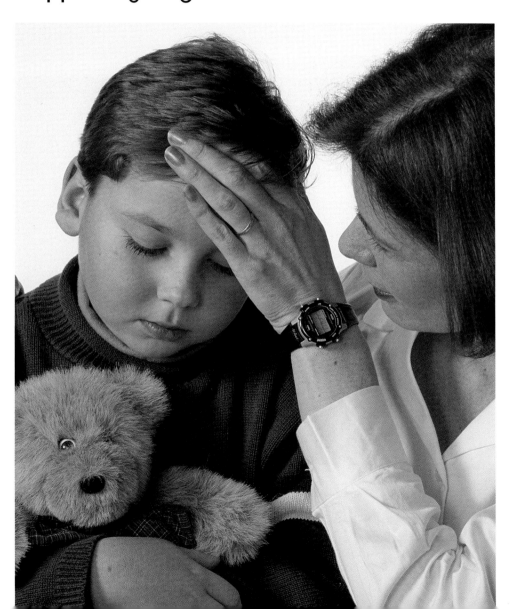

How Do You Catch It?

The whooping cough bacteria live in an **infected** person's nose, mouth, and throat. Whooping cough can spread when a person with whooping cough sneezes or coughs.

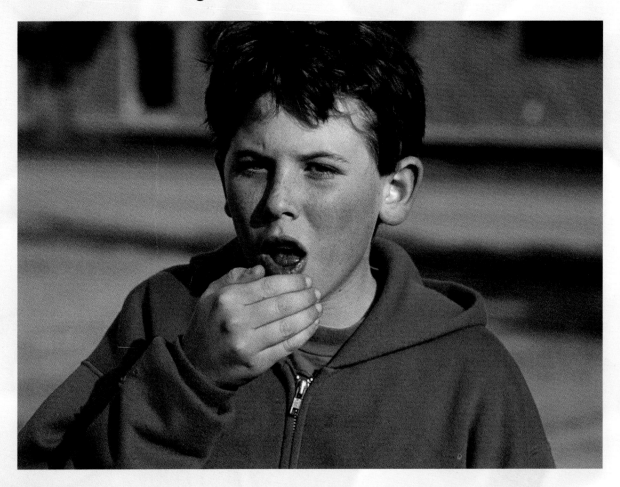

Sneezing and coughing send the whooping cough **bacteria** into the air. If you breathe in the bacteria, you may catch whooping cough.

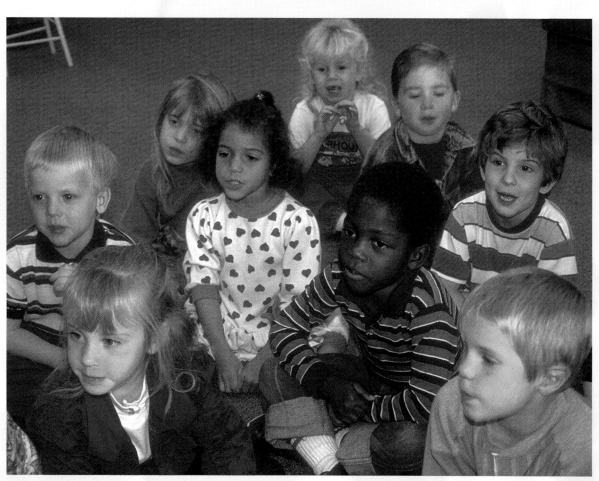

First Signs

The first signs of whooping cough are a lot like a cold. Your nose will run. You'll sneeze and have a little bit of a cough.

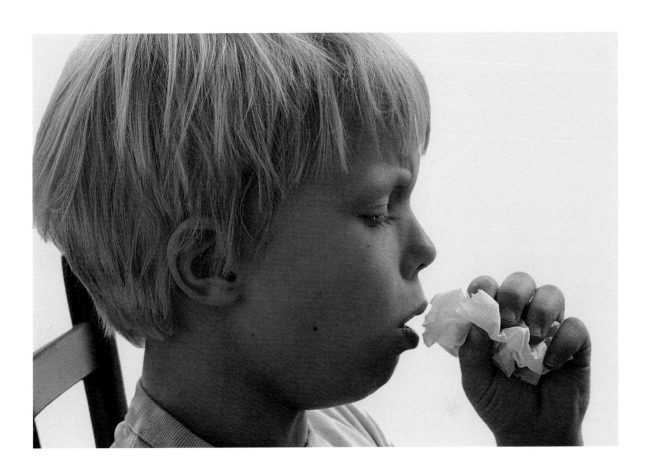

You may also have a **fever.** When you have a fever, your body's **temperature** is hotter than normal. This boy's mother is taking his temperature with a thermometer.

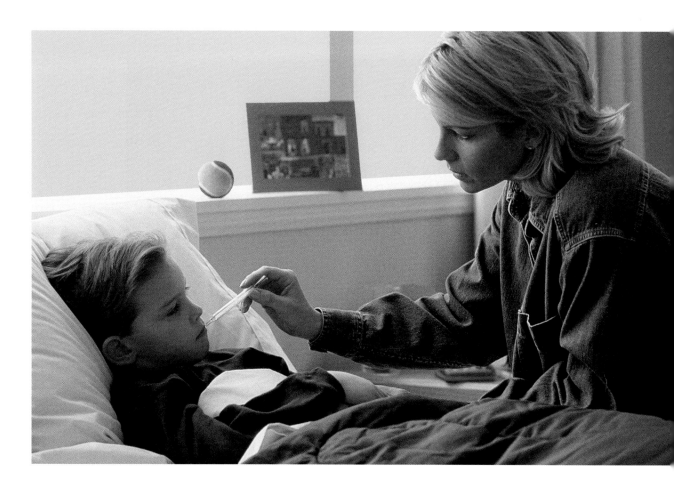

The Whooping Stage

In about a week or two, the cough gets worse. You may cough ten to twenty times in a row. This is called a **coughing fit.**

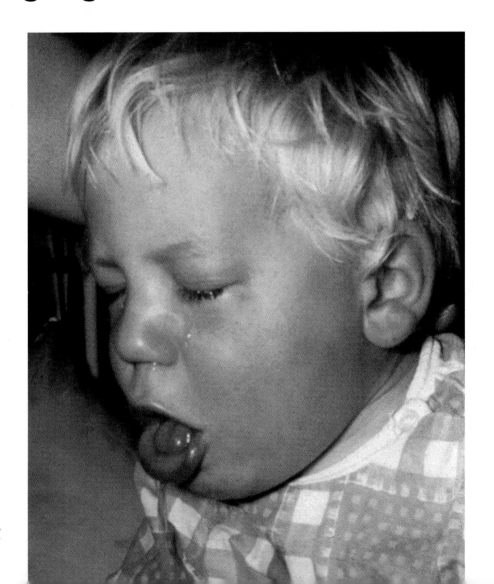

After the coughing fit ends, you will be very out of breath. You may make a "whooping" sound as you try to catch your breath.

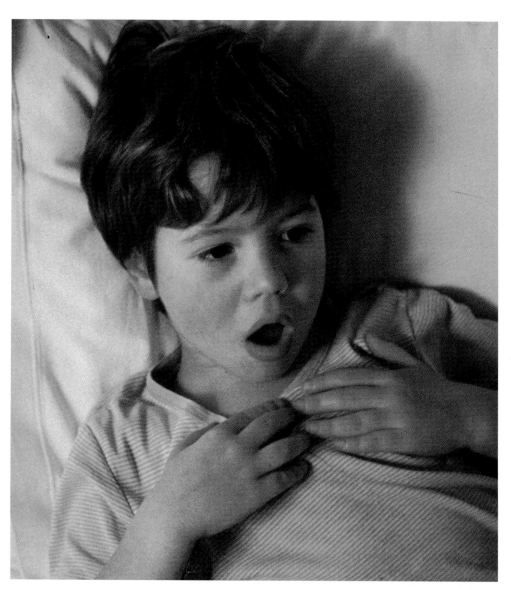

Why You Cough

The whooping cough **bacteria** cause your body to make a lot of **mucus.** This extra mucus builds up in your nose and **trachea.**

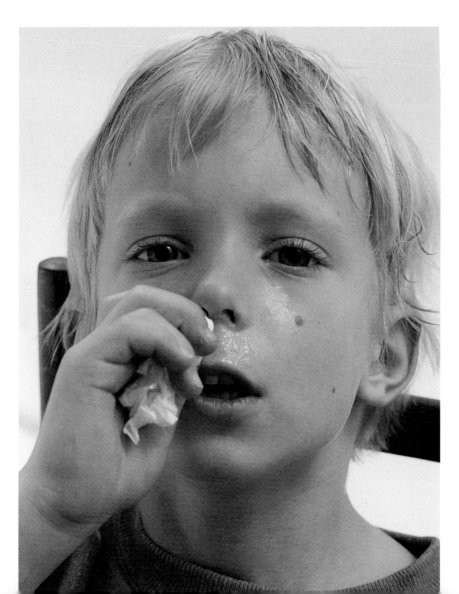

The **coughing fits** are how your body tries to clear out the mucus. Often during the coughing fits, you will cough up globs of mucus.

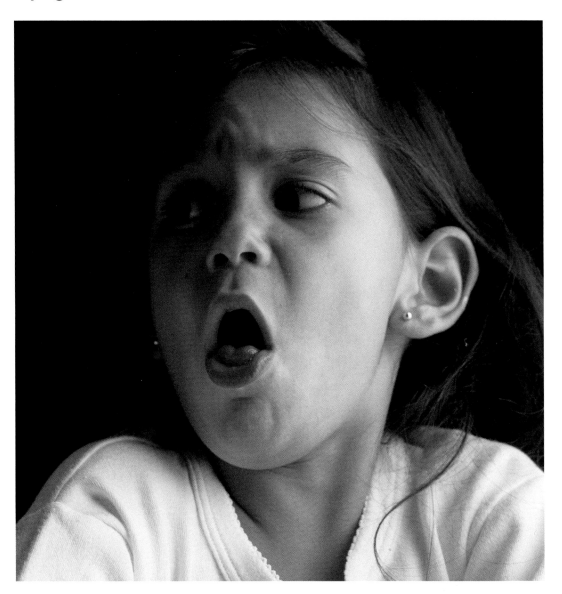

Treatment

If you have whooping cough, a doctor will give you **antibiotics.** Antibiotics are a kind of medicine that kills **bacteria.**

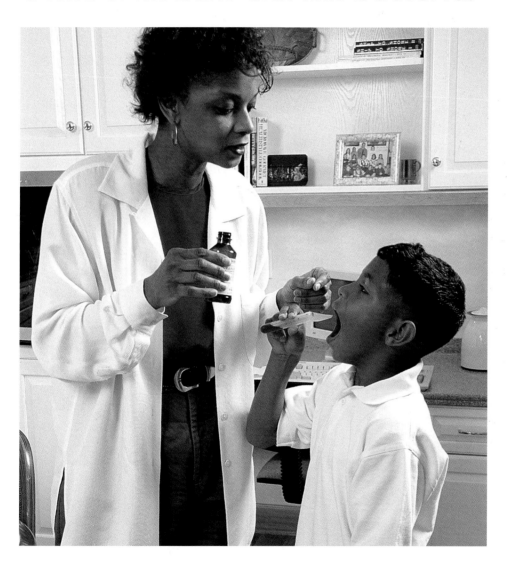

Because whooping cough is very **infectious,** everyone in your home will also have to take antibiotics. The antibiotics will help keep them from catching whooping cough from you.

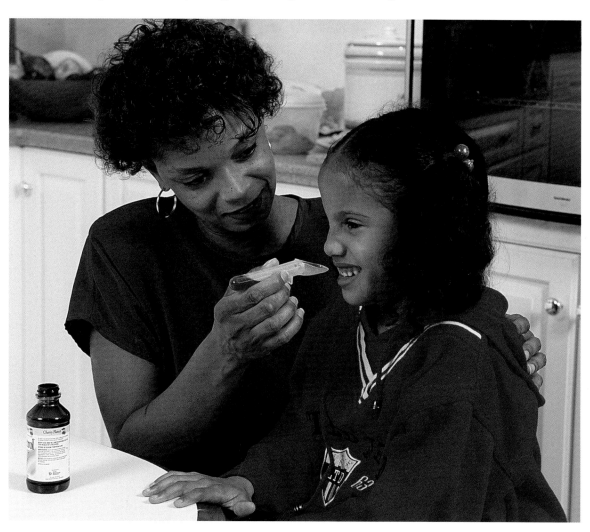

Whooping Cough Can Be Dangerous

If not treated, whooping cough can lead to a dangerous **infection** of the **lungs** called **pneumonia.** Whooping cough can be very serious for babies.

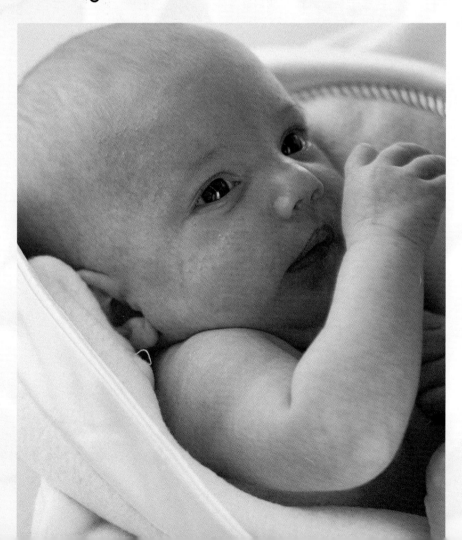

Young babies with whooping cough must go to the hospital. This way doctors can give the babies the care they need to keep whooping cough from getting worse.

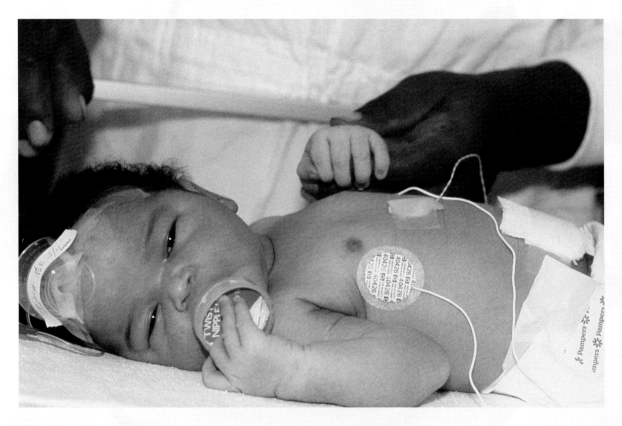

Getting Better

The **coughing fits** can last for three to four weeks. It may take even longer for you to feel well again.

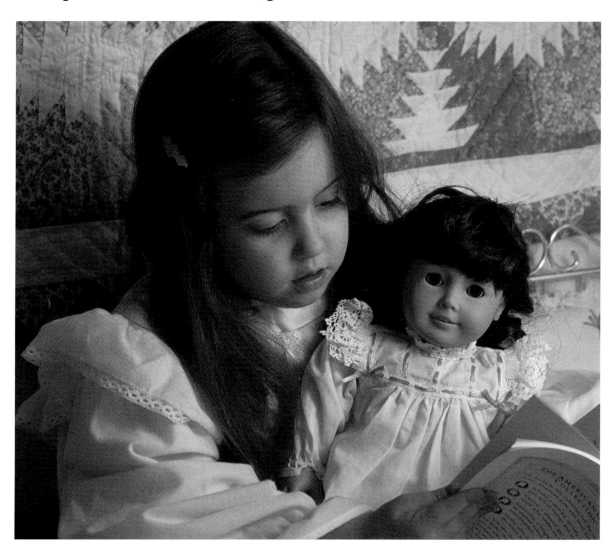

Your parents might put a **vaporizer** in your bedroom. The vaporizer will keep the air from getting too dry. It will help your body clear out **mucus.**

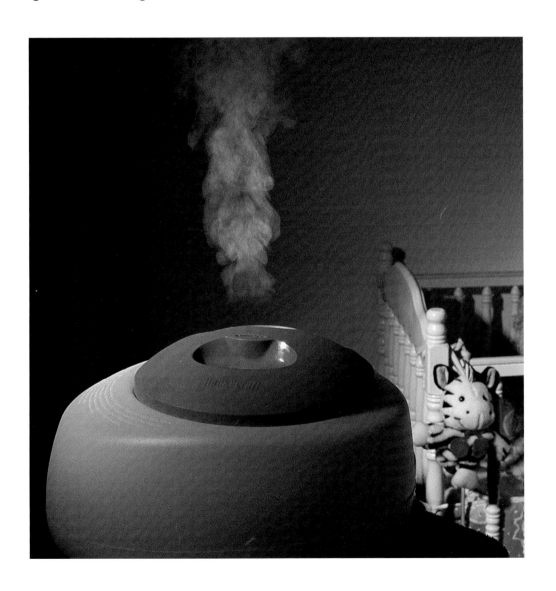

Avoiding Whooping Cough

People get a shot, or **vaccine,** that keeps them from getting whooping cough. Getting the vaccine gives people **immunity** to whooping cough. Babies get their first vaccine when they are about two months old.

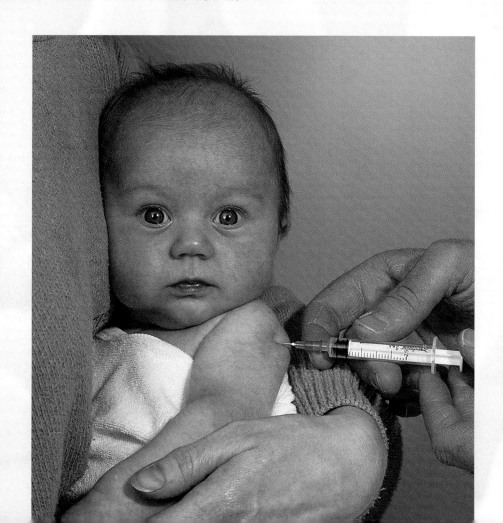

Children get three or four **booster shots** before they are five. Before the whooping cough vaccine was invented, many children got whooping cough. Today, whooping cough is less common.

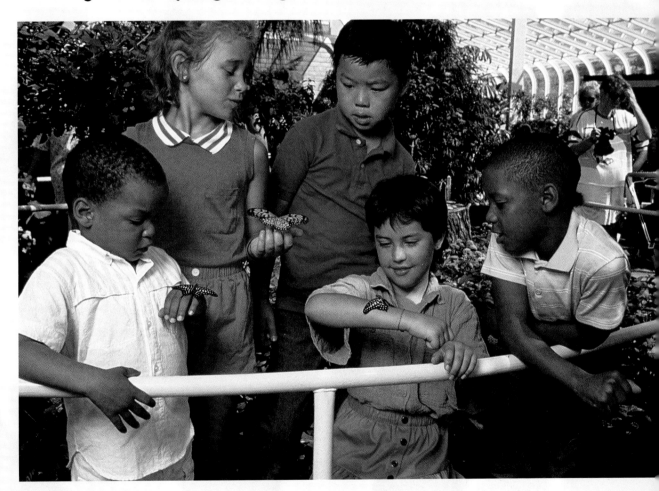

Staying Healthy

The whooping cough **vaccine** keeps most people from getting whooping cough. But it is still important to keep your body healthy.

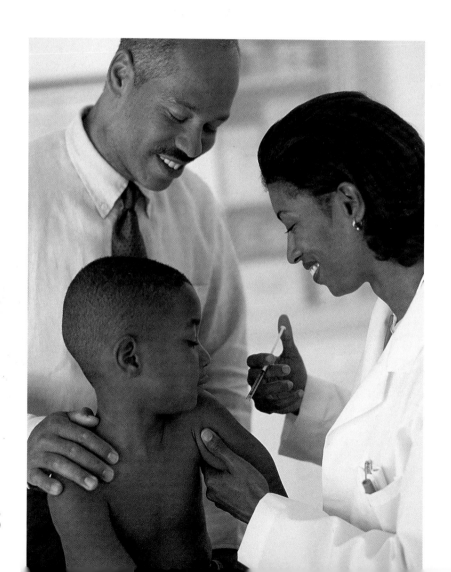

To stay strong and healthy, eat foods that are good for you. Get lots of exercise and get enough sleep. Wash your hands often to kill **germs** that might make you sick.

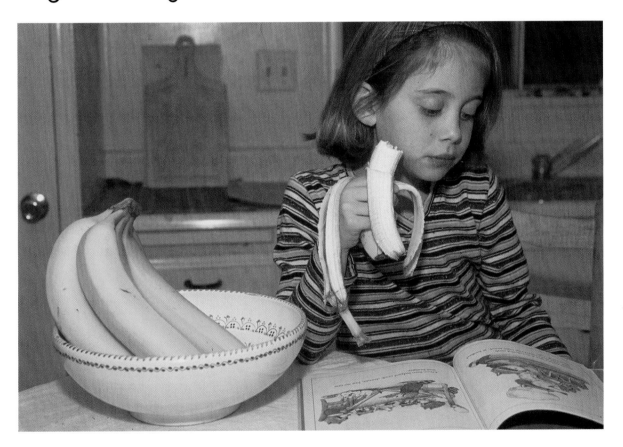

Think about It!

This baby has whooping cough. The doctor says the baby must go to the hospital. Why does the baby have to go to the hospital?*

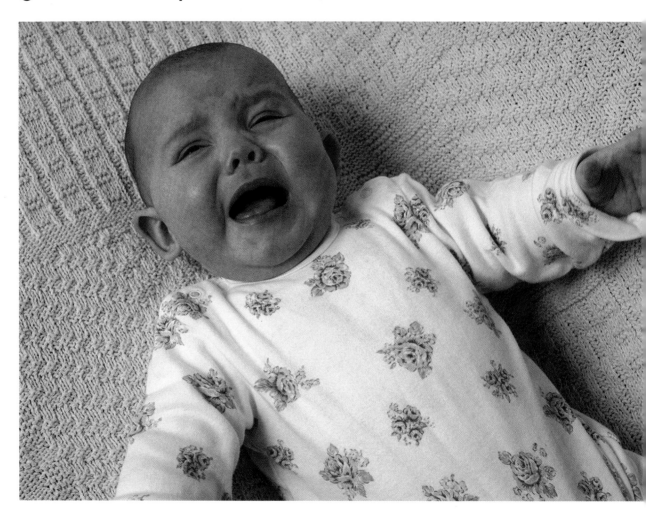

Rick's brother has whooping cough, but Rick does not. The doctor told him he must take **antibiotics** anyway. Why does the doctor want Rick to take antibiotics?*

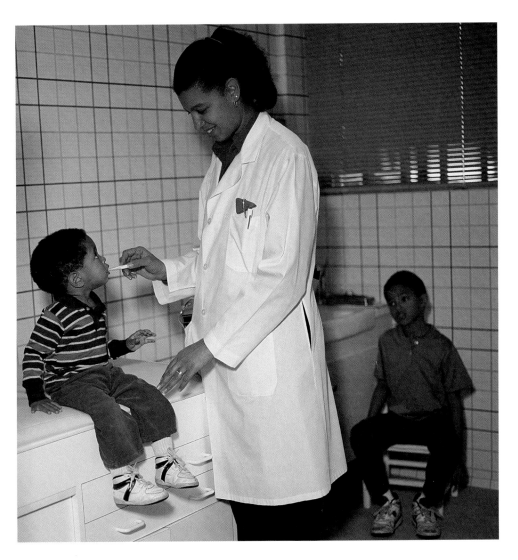

*Read page 30 to find out.

Answers

Page 28
Whooping cough can cause babies to get **pneumonia.**
At the hospital, doctors can give babies special care to
help them get better.

Page 29
Whooping cough is very **infectious.** The **antibiotics**
will help keep Rick from catching whooping cough from
his brother.

Stay Healthy and Safe!

1. Always tell an adult if you feel sick or think there
   is something wrong with you.

2. Never take any medicine unless it is given to you by
   an adult you trust.

3. Remember, the best way to stay healthy and safe
   is to eat good food, drink lots of water, keep clean,
   exercise, and get lots of sleep.

Glossary

antibiotics   medicine that kills bacteria

bacteria   tiny living things that can make you sick if they get in your body

booster shot   extra dose of vaccine given at a later time

coughing fit   coughing without stopping ten to twenty times in a row

fever   when the temperature of your body becomes hotter than usual

germ   tiny thing that can make you ill if it gets in your body

immunity   protection from getting an illness

infected   made sick or unhealthy by germs

infectious   can be passed from one person to another and can make you sick

lung   part of your body inside your chest that helps you breathe. People have two lungs.

microscope   machine that makes very small things look big enough to see

mucus   thick, sticky liquid that is inside your nose, throat, and lungs

pneumonia   type of dangerous lung infection

temperature   measure of how hot or cold something is

trachea   part of the throat that carries air to and from the lungs

vaccine   shot that keeps you from getting a sickness

vaporizer   machine that blows a cool mist of water into the air

Index

More Books to Read

Rowan, Kate. *I Know How We Fight Germs.* Cambridge, Mass.: Candlewick
    Press, 1999.

Royston, Angela. *Clean and Healthy.* Chicago: Heinemann Library, 1999.

Saunders-Smith, Gail. *The Doctor's Office.* Minnetonka, Minn.: Capstone
    Press, 1998.